Alkaline Anti – inflammatory Diet

A Guide to Detoxifying, Healthy Life and Vitality

Lionel Chris

Disclaimer

Kindly note. the information contained in this document is for general purposes only. You should not rely on this material or information in this book as the basis for making any decisions without the adequate knowledge and contribution of experts. While the writer endeavours to keep the information up to date and correct, the writer makes no representations or warranties of any kind,

Dedication

This book is dedicated to everyone facing one health challenge or the other.

Table of Contents

Alkaline Anti – inflammatory Diet 1

Dedication 4

Introduction 8

Chapter 1 10

What is alkaline 10

CHAPTER 2 13

What is Inflammation? 13

Chapter 3 17

What is a diet? 17

Chapter 4 30

Alkaline Foods and Drinks...................................30

Chapter 5 50

Alkaline Diet 50

Chapter 6 54

Acidic Diets...................................54

Chapter 7 59

Making The Body More Alkaline 59

About The Author 63

Acknowledgement..64

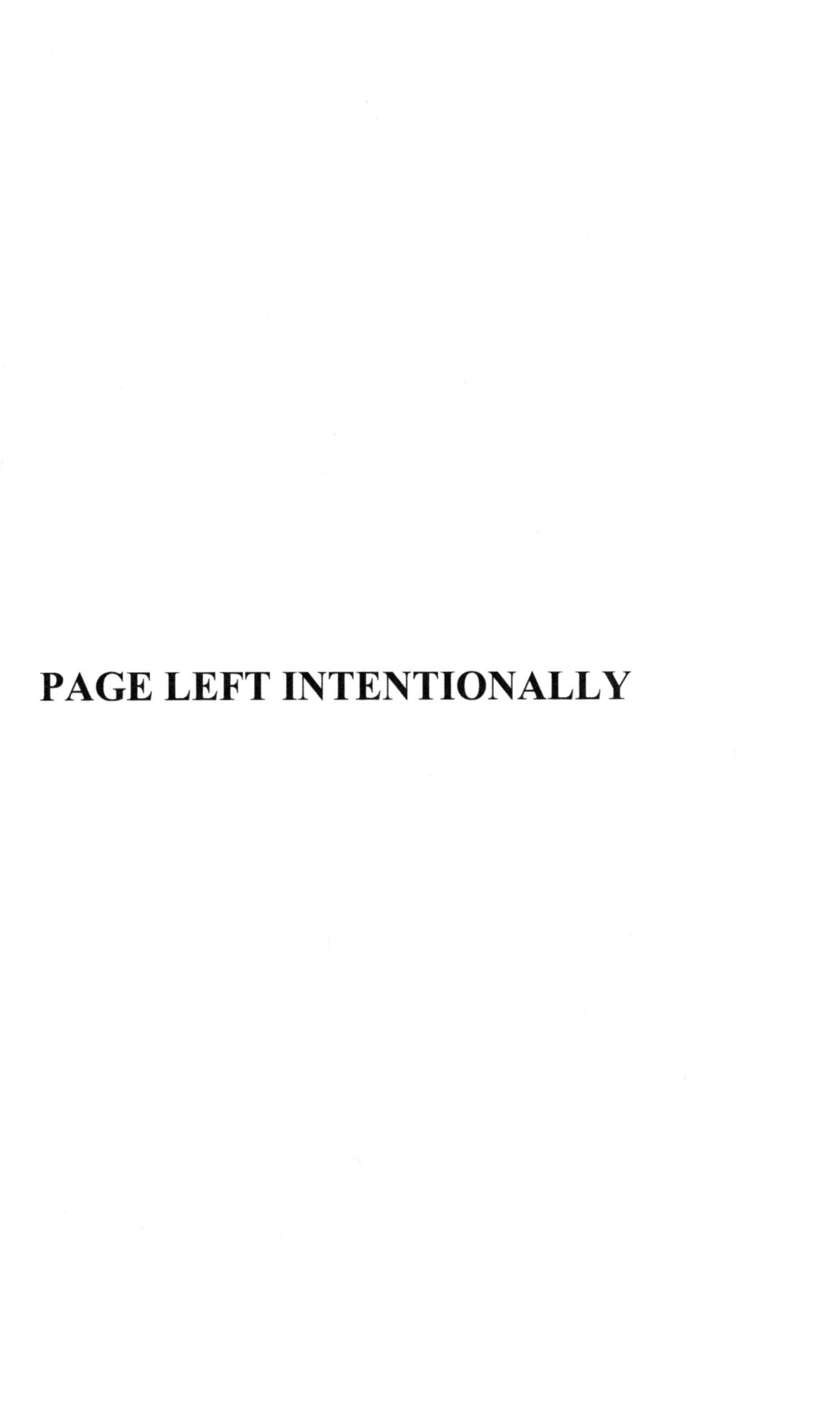

PAGE LEFT INTENTIONALLY

Introduction

Nurturing an acidic body is a dangerous experience too risky. Nevertheless, it can be worked on by deliberately filling the body with substances that combat this. An alkali body will ensure that the body immune system works appropriately. Thus, this book expatiates on what the body needs to be alkaline and:

- ✓ What alkaline diet is

- ✓ The available different diets.

- ✓ pH level.

- ✓ Neutral pH

- ✓ What the body needs to be alkali.

- ✓ Inflammation

- ✓ Types of inflammation

- ✓ Alkaline in relation to inflammatory

- ✓ Seasonal foods

✓ Nuts.

✓ The diets for alkaline

…and many more.

After reading this book, you will know what pH stands for and the effects of acidity and alkaline consumption in the body.

Chapter 1

What is alkaline

A substance can either be acidic or alkaline based on the pH level.

pH level helps to determine the acidic or alkalinity of substance using the scale of 0 to 14. that is either acidic or alkaline to determine this. Any substance that the pH is 0 is completely considered acidic while any substance that the pH is considered very alkaline. The pH level of some substances can be 7 which can be considered neutral. With the body system, the alkaline level varies all through ranging between 7.35pH level and 7.45pH level. Alkaline (that is alkaline water) is believed to have the ability to neutralize the acid in the body because it has higher pH level than the ordinary drinking water which falls within the categories of pH neutral level, that is 7pH whereas alkaline water has as much as 8pH/9pH level.

What does 'Alkaline' mean?

A neutral pH (potential of Hydrogen) of 7.4 on a scale of 0 to 14, is where the body functions best. On the pH scale, 0-7 is acidic, while 7-14 is alkaline. The foods we eat are broken down into acid and alkaline, and broadly speaking, most people lean towards being acidic, based on eating more acidic food than alkaline. This doesn't relate to the food itself, for example, lemons are acidic but are actually digested by the body to have an alkalising effect. It is highly postulated by health professionals that high acidity poses dangerous threat to the body. It depletes vital body resources thereby weakening the roles of the body systems as well as bringing about inflammation. Acidic diet come with hurting joints, gaining weight, craving for sugar and / or carb, and brain fog. An alkaline diet is rich in vegetables and fruit, herbs, soybeans and tofu – more plants, less animal products.

It is advisable to have more negative ORP value. ORP which stands for Oxidation Reduction Potential is described as the ability of water to perform as a pro- or antioxidant. This must be contained in alkaline water alongside alkaline minerals and negative ORP.

Naturally, alkaline water has pH of 8 or 9. Nevertheless, only pH is not sufficient to make water substantially alkalinised.

CHAPTER 2

What is Inflammation?

For the purpose of this topic, here is a brief description of inflammation.

Inflammation can be simply described as the body defence system where the body makes a protective attempt to fight and remove harmful stimuli. If not for inflammatory body responses, wounds will not heal up, damages to tissues cannot be repaired and infections will not be combated. In other words, inflammation aids healings.

Is inflammation painful?

The answer is yes following these explanations. How severe inflammation determines the pain to feel. There could be such pains as agony, discomfort, distress, stiffness, etc. which can be constant and steady, pulsating and throbbing, stabbing or pinching. Signals are sent to the brain when unfriendly activities happen to the body. The brain sends it back after passing through some processes in the body which results in pains.

Other biochemical processes also occur during inflammation. They affect how nerves work, and this can heighten pain. When inflammation lingers for longer time, it often leads to pain as it causes more harms to the body.

Types of Inflammation

There are basically two types of inflammation namely Acute and Chronic.

Acute Inflammation

Inflammation is said to be acute when in a short space of time it becomes severe starting rapidly. The symptoms of acute inflammation are usually noticed for few days but may, in some cases, continue for few weeks. The following diseases experiences can result in acute inflammation – acute bronchitis, acute appendicitis, dermatitis, high-intensity exercise, infected ingrown toenail, infective meningitis, physical trauma, sore throat, scratch / cut on the skin, sinusitis, tonsillitis, etc.

Chronic Inflammation

On the other hand, chronic inflammation lasts for a longer time than acute inflammation. While acute can last for just weeks, chronic inflammation lasts for months and may be years. This could be as a result of acute inflammation advancing to chronic inflammation because of neglect or haphazard treatment or attention. It can also be as a result of mistaking autoimmune for disease causing pathogens thereby attacking healthy tissue. There is also the exposure to industrial chemical which can cause irritant for a long period of time. Active hepatitis, asthma, chronic peptic ulcer, periodontitis, rheumatoid arthritis, sinusitis, tuberculosis (TB), ulcerative colitis, hay fever, etc are example of diseases and conditions that can be described as chronic inflammation.

Chapter 3

What is a diet?

Diet may be described as the habitual consumption of substance (food) by a person, an animal or group of persons. It can also be described as a special course or quantity of feeding, food or consumption to which a person restricts or places self.

Dieting could be based on health reasons or other reasons like weight management or control, ethical, religions and beliefs.

Different Kinds of diets

As earlier mentioned that diet / dieting can be based on several factors, we shall make a list of some available kinds of diets as it relates to some factors.

Belief based Diet

This type of diet is attached to religion, spiritual and / philosophical idea and opinion. You may want to carry out more research on this.

Calories and Weight management/control Diets

This diet is based on decision to lose or gain/add weight. That is weight control. Weight can be control either by adding to it or by shedding. For this to be achievable, focus and attention must be placed on what is taken-in in form of food and drinks. We consider diets like LOW CALORIES DIETS under this topic.

Maintaining a particular weight puts into consideration the carefully monitoring of calories that is consumed

Low Calories Diets

Having less than 1200 calories per day as an adult is an example of diet on low calories. It is consisting of fewer calories than needed to sustain weight. It also looks at rationing of fats, protein and carbohydrates.

Low Carbohydrate Diet

This is also geared towards weight loss observing four phases of induction, balancing, fine-tuning and maintenance. It involves the steady and regular increase in consumption of carbohydrate.

Some experts are of the opinion that dieting for weight loss is not completely cutting off carbohydrates but taking it in a particularly advised quantity.

Low Fat Diets

This is otherwise known as starch diet. It is premised on the consumption of foods that are starchy in components e.g beans, potatoes, rice, etc.

Crash Diets

Crash diets is a very dangerous diet as it can lead to death if not well observed and not in accordance with professional advice and recommendation. The changes made on food to eat under crash diet has to be rapid and extreme.

Cabbage Soup Diet

This is another low calories diet plan. It is heavily based on cabbage soup consumption. Cabbage soup is a soup that is made from carrots, celery, onions, cabbage, diced tomato and spices.

Grapefruit Diet

This falls under fad diet. It is a method of weight loss diet that is based on the consumption of grapefruits in large quantities during meal time.

Monotrophic Diet

As the prefix "mono" implies, this postulate the consumption of one type of food for a period of time in order to achieve desired result of weight control – reduction.

Detox Diets

Detoxifying is the process of removing unhealthy substances from the body. This is observed by refraining from taking some foods or drinks. In like strain, consuming some foods or / and some drinks help in this regard. Taking water at a particular time of the day and the quantity taken is considered detoxification to some extent.

Juice Fasting

This is also another form of detox diet. It is a form of nutrition obtained mainly from fruits and vegetables via juicing.

Diets Allowed for Medical Reasons

Dieting can be based on professional medical advice. Because of the effects of some consumption which can be beneficial where a reduction or addition is, or for some other reasons, some pattern of dieting can be recommended and administered in order to subject the patient to self-discipline and to achieve desired results.

Diet for Hypertension

This is a diet based on the recommendation of medical experts. Persons with high blood pressure are placed on diet where they are to consume fruits, vegetables, wholegrains, low fat dairy foods in large quantities. This recommendation also includes avoidance of sugar, sweetened foods, red meat.

Gluten-free Diet

Some disorderliness are gluten related. For this, it is professionally advised to avoid protein gluten. This type of protein can be found in barley, rye and wheat.

Healthy Kidney Diet

While this does not in any way represent kidney dialysis, it is a medical advice for persons with kidney problems whether kidney failure, chronic kidney disease, single kidney or kidney infectious persons. Under this diet, because it is often hard to be broken down, consumption of large amount of protein is restricted. This is to be taken in limited quantity.

Ketogenic Diet

This diet is popular for its usage as a medical treatment for refractory epilepsy. It converts body fat into energy. It is also known to be of high fat, adequate protein and a low carbohydrate diet.

Egg and Wine Diet

This is a diet that is drafted in observation of the daily menu of breakfast, lunch and dinner. For breakfast menu – one egg and a glass of white wine, for lunch – two eggs and glass of wine and for dinner – steak and what is left of the wine.

Food Combining Diet

Where, for example, protein given foods and carbohydrates foods are deliberately consumed together or separately, this implies food combining diet.

Fit for Life Diet

This is a diet where it is recommended not to combine some classes of food i.e protein and carbohydrate, waiting till after meal time before drinking water, and refraining from eating dairy foods.

Zone Diet

Is described as a diet in which attempt is made at splitting the intake of calorie from carbohydrates, protein and fats in a particular proportion.

Pritikin Diet

Under this diet, there is focus on the consumption of unprocessed food.

Vegetarian Diet

This is a diet in which consumption is based on mainly vegetables. This diet rejects meat and by-products of slaughtered animals.

Lacto Vegetarian

This diet is mostly religious base. It prevents the consumption of eggs and foods that contain animal rennet

Ovo Vegetarianism

The word ovo is a Latin word for egg. It is a type of vegetarianism which allows for the consumption of eggs but not dairy products.

Ovo – Lacto Vegetarianism

This is the direct contrast of ovo vegetarianism in that it allows for the consumption of both eggs and dairy products.

Vegan Diet

This is diet goes beyond just consumption. Aside from separating self from the consumption of any substance that is a bye product of animal, those on this diet protects the right of animals by speaking against cruelty to animals and animal's exploitations for consumption or any other production. This is in addition to their abstaining from a vegetarian diet and includes not using products that are of animals e.g egg, dairy products, honey, etc

Fruitarian Diet

Predominantly, this diet consists of consumption of raw fruits.

Low Carb Diet

This diet is presupposed on losing weight by restricting carbohydrates.

Alkaline Diet

This is the avoidance of acidic food, that is food that have low pH level. Examples of such foods are alcohol, caffeine, dairy, fungi, grains, glucose and meat.

High Protein Diet

This is targeted at muscles building. It advocates for consumption of high quantities of protein.

High Residue Diet

Is that diet that concentrates on the consumption of high quantities of dietary fibre. This food includes certain fruits, vegetables, nuts and grains.

Organic Food Diet

We are at present in the world or processed foods which implies that such produce may have been produced with synthetic fertilizer, genetic modifications, and / or additives. Organic food diet preaches the consumption of foods that ensures the absence of any and all of the above mentioned food processing substances.

Ray Food Diet

This consists of the consumption of foods that have not been cooked and processed. This is also common with people who practice vegetarian as diet.

Sugar Buster

This is a diet where there is restriction on the consumption of refined carbohydrate, in particular, sugar.

For further varieties of diets, visit the web.

Chapter 4

Alkaline Foods and Drinks

Mentioned below are some foods that have alkaline

Lemonade

Because lemons, as an excellence of Vitamin C, are also great sources of folate and potassium, it is traditionally packed with sugar and is alkalinized. A drink with a slice of lemon makes the drink healthier.

Coconut Water

Coconut water drink is a naturally sweetened drink filled with Vitamin C, Calcium, Dietary fibre and Riboflavin.

This is a recommendable drink for any athletes' recovery from the energy burnt as a result of exercises because of the presence of electrolytes and sodium.

Ginger Herbal Tea

This is an alkaline drink that can be enjoyed either hot or cold. Adding slice of ginger or making ginger tea straight away makes a perfect healthy tea. With a ginger based drink, there is an assurance of a relive from problems such as indigestive, loss of appetite, motion sickness, and nausea. It also helps to reduce the risk of diabetes, heart disease and obesity.

Alkaline Water

Filtering out contaminants which include aluminium, chlorine, copper and lead, one can say a mineralized water is the healthiest drink that can be. This is because of the presence of pH balanced water.

Spinach

Findings have shown that spinach is an essential consumption with vitamins and minerals. The vitamins found in spinach include vitamins A, C, E, K and Vitamin B6. It is an alkaline-forming loaded consumption with folate, calcium, iron and magnesium but with a very little saturated fats and cholesterol. Spinach is a source of niacin, fibre and protein. Based on studies, it is said to be an antioxidant that helps to fights different kinds of cancer. It has healthy benefits for bones because it contains calcium.

Kale

Kale also have nutritional benefits as other leafy substances and high in alkaline contents. A glass of kale 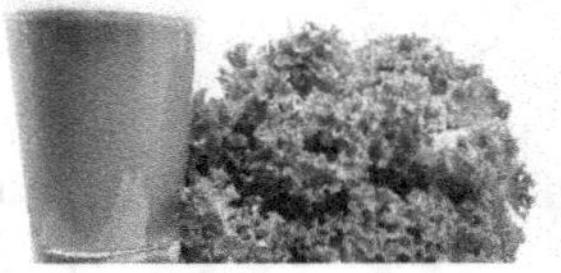 drink gives more than 100% needed daily vitamin A, vitamin C and a very huge value of vitamin K. A cup of kale drinks contains enzyme sulforaphane which also keeps cancer and other illnesses away.

Cucumber

Cucumber is a combination of vitamins 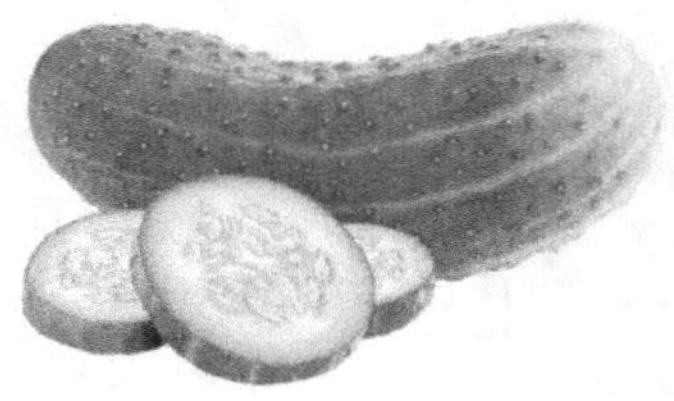 and minerals. These two help to neutralize acid in the body while alkaline is sustained. Cucumber is a great source of consumption because of the presence of some phytonutrients e.g lignans and flavonoids. The benefits of the phytonutrients include anti-inflammatory and anti-cancer. Cucumber is mostly water hence dehydrates.

Broccoli

Containing numerous vitamins such as vitamin C, vitamin K and minerals e.g folate, manganese and iron broccoli helps to neutralize acid in the body. One of the

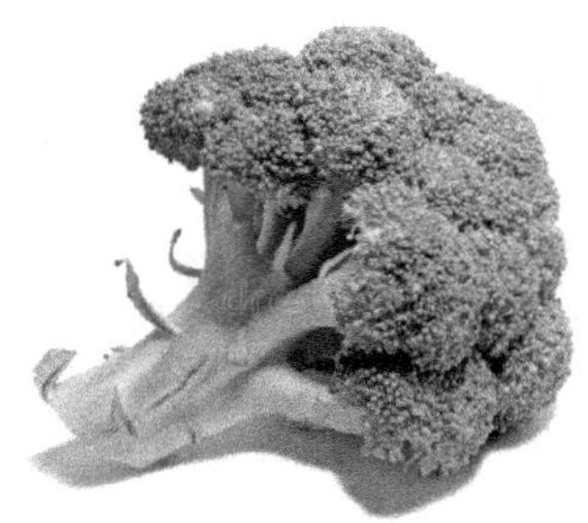

properties of broccoli that helps in effectively protecting against various types of cancer is the sulforaphane. Broccoli is also known for helping to aid healthy eye as well as lower cholesterol level.

Avocado

Avocado is a great source of monounsaturated fatty acids (e.g oleic acid). Avocado is another alkaline consumable. It is nutritious and helps to reduce inflammation, heart 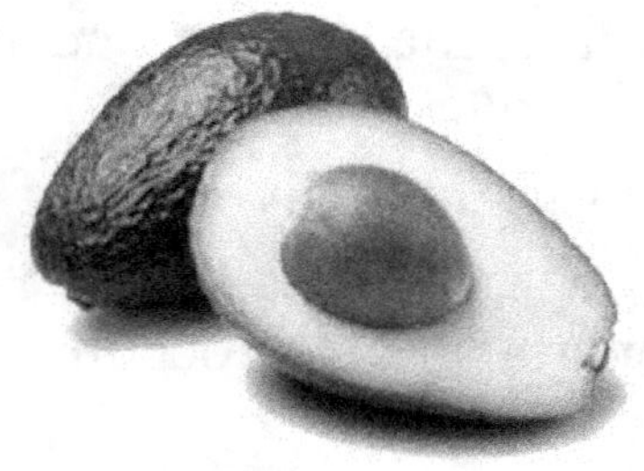 disease, and helps prevents cancer. Avocado like other foods mentioned above contains folate which is necessary for healthy cell functioning and tissue growth, vitamin k needed to aid healthy bone, potassium for alkalizing mineral essential and copper needed for healthy heart.

Celery

Celery is highly antioxidant and has enzymes that are beneficial. As it is with other alkaline solution, a host of

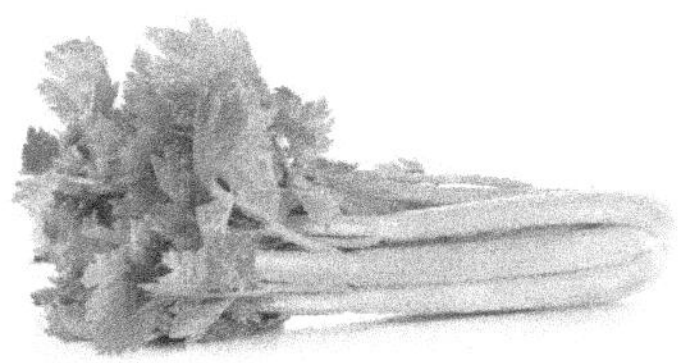

similar vitamins, minerals and potassium are found in a glass cupful of a celery drink that aids alkalizing and fights inflammatory. Present in celery are vitamin C, vitamin K, vitamin B6, potassium, its water content is astronomical and significant fibre content. Among other benefits, one stands to achieve easy digestion and weight loss.

Sprouts

This is another source of vitamins and minerals. Very high in calcium magnesium,

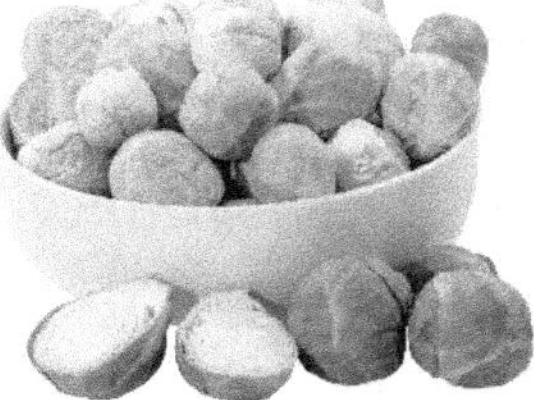

potassium, iron and zinc all needed for neutralizing acidity but replenishing mineral stores in the body. Sprouts contain resources needed for preventing cancer and protecting DNA which as a result of the presence of chlorophyll which is also part of alkaline minerals.

GREEN LEAFY VEGETABLES

There are some essentials minerals required by the body to perform and carry out some functions. Green leafy vegetables include argula, celery, kale, lettuce, mustard green, parsley, spinach, etc.

Cauliflower

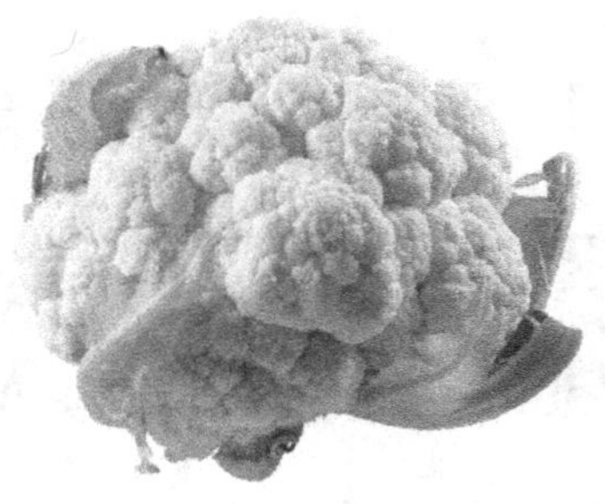

Cauliflower comprises of a nutrient that regulates the levels of estrogen in the body when this becomes too high. Estrogen is a body compound that we come in contact with through the consumption of some foods such as soy, chemicals such as plastics and pharmaceuticals drugs such as oral contraceptives. This estrogen are harmful to the body as it can give way to gaining weight, bloating, reproductive cancer and infertility. Cauliflower being an alkaline food can help in aiding rebalancing of hormones in combating estrogen in the body

CITRUS FRUITS

Contrary to a lay man perspective of citrus fruits being highly acidic, this is among the best sources of alkaline foods and consumption. Among citrus fruits are lemon, lime and oranges which are loaded with Vitamin C and are identified to aid detoxifying the body system and providing relieves from acidity and heart burn.

Seaweeds

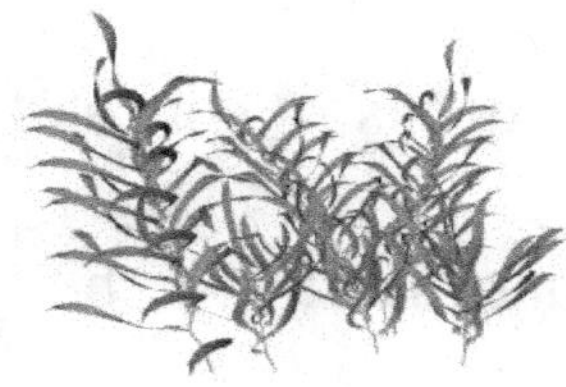 Seaweed (or sea vegetables) are study proven to contain 10-12 times more mineral content than those grown on land. They are also believed to be high source of alkaline.

Swiss Chard

This a family of green with adequate nutrition benefits 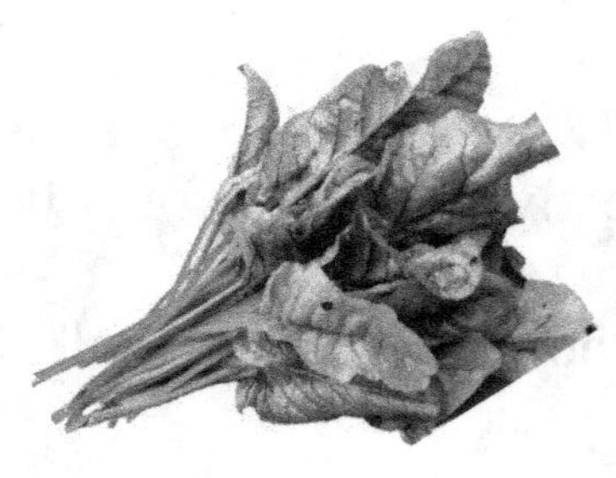 with vitamins that support healthy cell e.g vitamin k. When it is metabolised, Swiss chard increased alkalizing minerals than acidity.

ROOT VEGETABLES

Root Vegetables are great sources of alkali some of which are best tasted when spiced-roasted. These alkalizing foods include sweet potato, taro root, lotus root, beets and carrots.

Beets

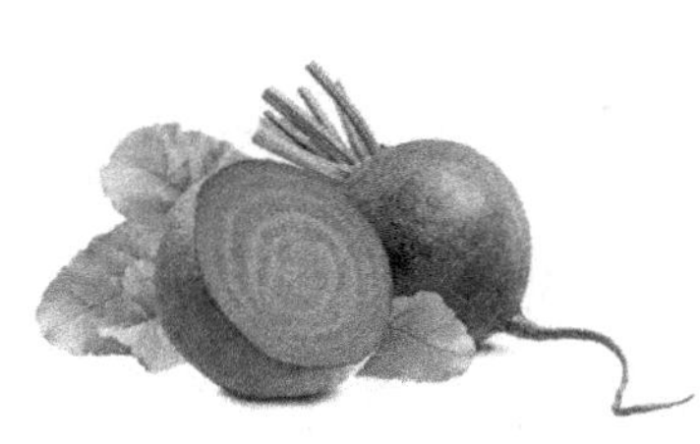

Beets are considered the world's most alkaline food. Beets bitter quality is an addition in that, for better fats digestion, this may help to stimulate bile production.

Carrot

Carrot is famous for its vitamin A content good for improving eyesight.

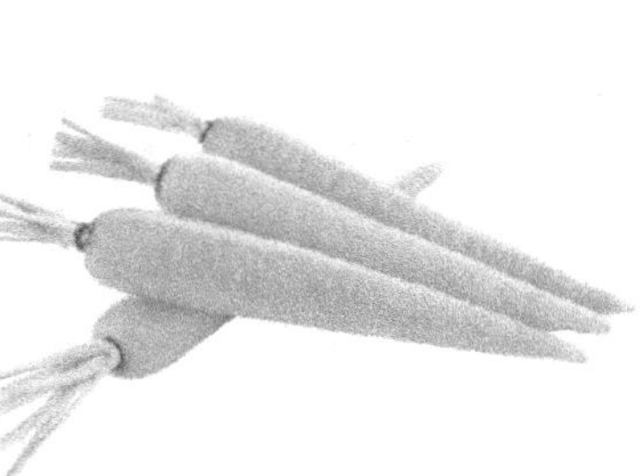

Its contents include beta-carotene which is an antioxidant and hich can also help work on the skin.

Sweet Potato

The best tasted sweet potato is the fried and spiced one. This is unarguably starchy but it is a rich alkali and provides the body with fibre, minerals and vitamins. 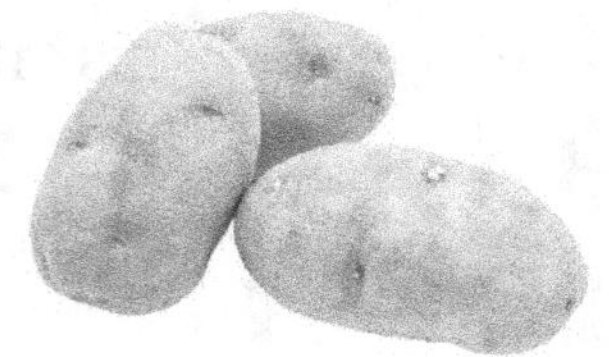 Being fibre in nature, its sweetened feature does not portend danger to the body because fibre helps to slow the release of sugar into the blood stream. It can therefore be described as an excellent food in that it gives energy to the body and it is alkalinizing.

SEASONAL FRUITS

Nutritionists and other related experts have postulated that taking seasonal fruits in a daily diet can be beneficial to health. Seasonal fruits have been proven to contain vitamins, minerals and antioxidants that performs numerous roles in the body and are very high sources of alkaline. They include kiwi, pineapple, persimmon, nectarine, watermelon, grapefruit, apricots and apples.

kiwi

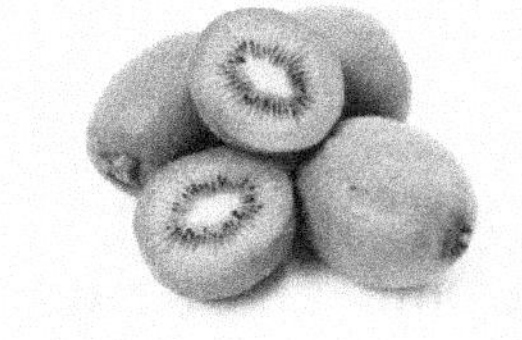

Kiwi is an alkaline food. It is an antioxidants food and contains vitamins and minerals in notable high quantity. It contains more vitamin C than orange is known to contain. All of these aid improved digestion plus potassium needed for improved muscles functioning.

Pineapple

Pineapple is known to aid digestion. It is an alkalizing foods that contains bromelain which 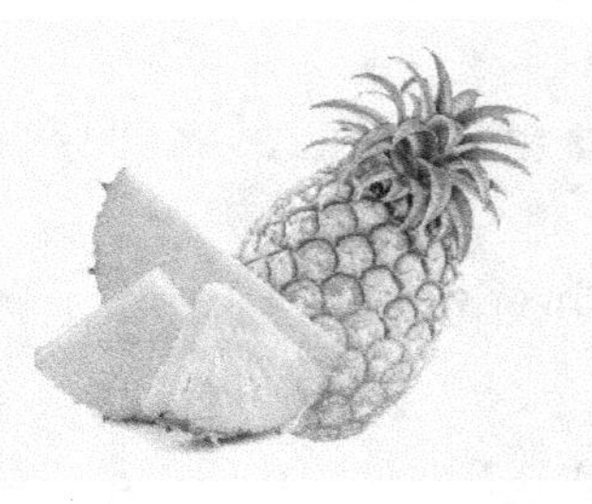 is claimed to be helpful in killing parasites that are found in the intestine. Bromelain are digestive enzymes and can stand as the reason for the digestive feature of a pineapple.

Watermelon

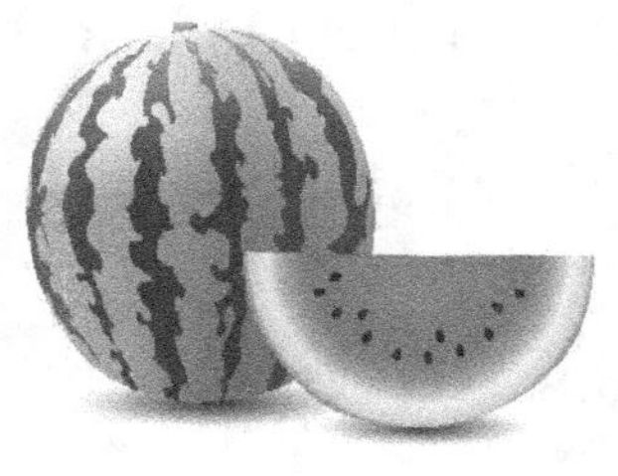 An electrolyte and alkalizing foods almost 100% liquid, watermelon is essential for cardiac function, dehydration, detoxification, anti-inflammatory, etc.

Apples

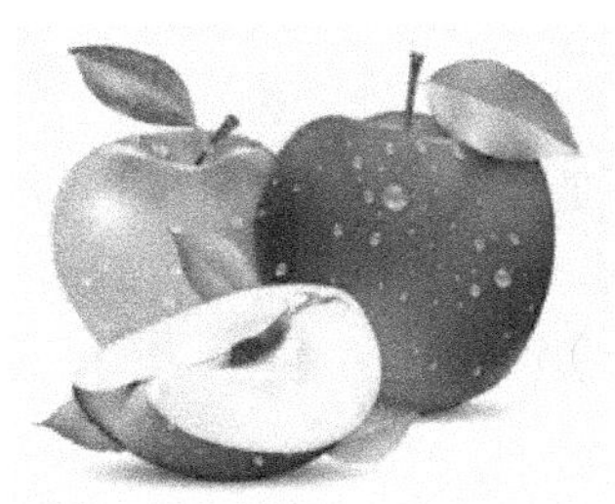

This a globally rated food as the healthiest food. This is largely depended on its richly fibre contents for which it detoxifies, vitamin C to act as antioxidant, and flavonoids for the protection against cancer; Every nutrient needed to promote healthy blood pressure and cholesterol.

Persimmons

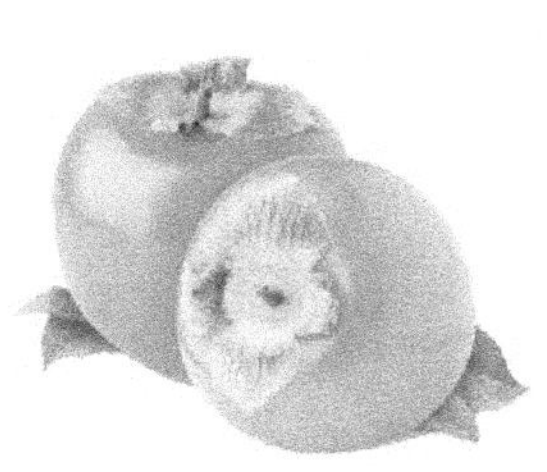

Persimmon contains many health promoting phytonutrients examples of which are catechin and gallocatechin both of which are antioxidants. It is fibre and also contains betulinic acid which has been argued to have antiretroviral, antimalarial, and is also anti-inflammatory. Other nutrients are manganese, beta-carotene, vitamin C and iron. Persimmons are anticancer agent.

Nectarine

Nectarine are of different colours namely white, yellow, orange and red. This is also seen on their pulp. Nectarine is a load of many health benefits that include vitamin A, vitamin C, potassium and antioxidants nutrient.

Grapefruits

Grapefruit is known to be source of vitamins and other

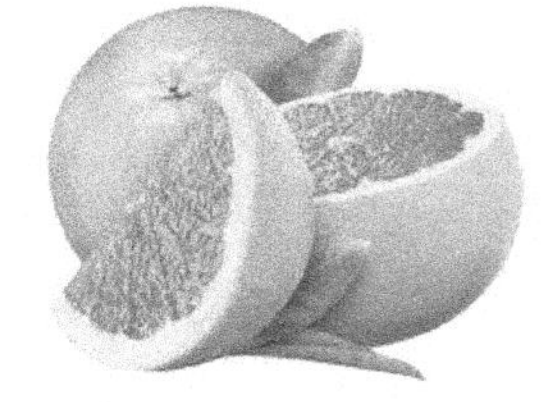 nutrients. Grapefruit is categorised as fibre and it is an antioxidant helping to boost immunity. It aids digestion and lowering of cholesterol. Other nutritional value of grapefruit includes vitamins A and C, folate (B9), choline, limonins and lycopene. It aids weight loss.

Apricots

Apricots are fruits rich in vitamin A also known as retinol. It is a soluble which helps in vision 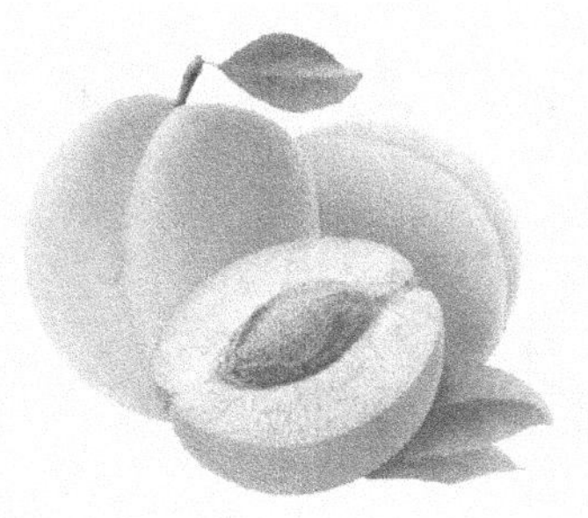 enhancement as well as keeping the immune system in form while protecting the skin. In fact, it helps reduce the chances of loss of vision as a result of the presence of retinol and beta-carotene. Fatty acids are broken down which implies that digestion are well taken care of consuming apricots. It helps cleans intestine regularly protecting gastrointestinal worries. Like every other fibre meal, it helps to reduce cholesterols content in the body protecting the heart. It is a natural sources of antioxidants getting rid of toxins.

Banana

Banana, known as potassium stick, is a great source of fibre which promotes digestive regularity. It helps strikes out 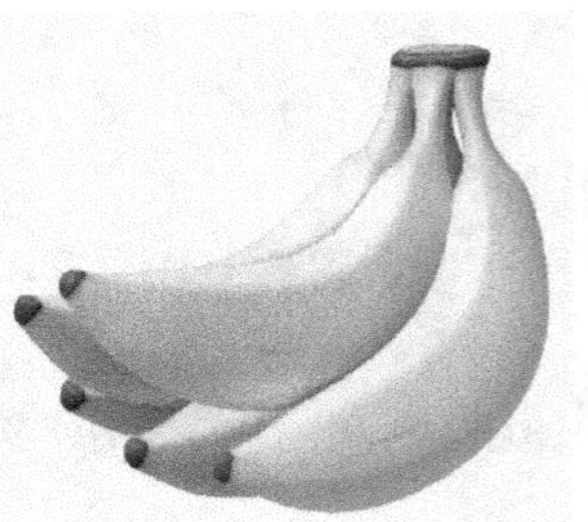 toxins from the gastrointestinal tract. Banana is highly alkalinized.

NUTS

These are alkaline producing foods substances that are highly in calories. They are also a good sources of fats which is the why it is advised to be consumed in limited quantity. They include cashews, chestnuts and almonds.

Cashew

Cashew are said to be rich in fatty acids for healthy heart. Consumption of cashews may help increase your iron levels which could be beneficial to your immune system. Cashews are also known to be a source of copper providing minerals. The percentage of copper produced by cashews are of recommended daily intake which may help to reduce the risk of chronic diseases.

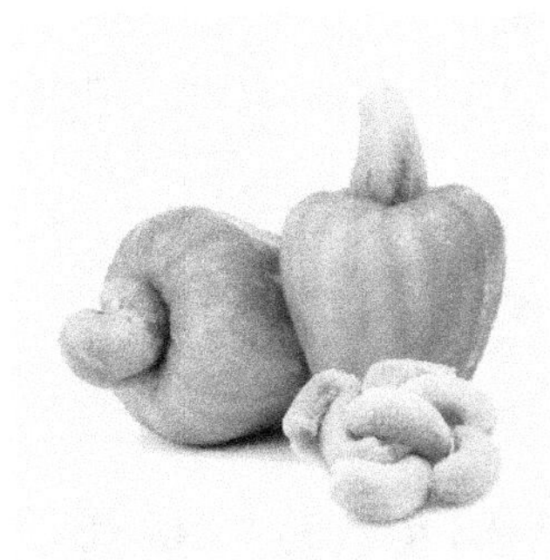

Almond

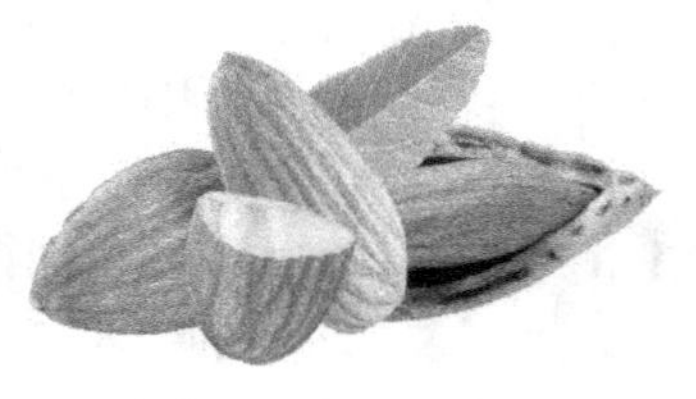

In whatever way of either raw or toasted, almonds contain a good volume of daily needed protein. Almonds are rich in vitamin, minerals, protein and fibre. It helps lower overall level of cholesterol. Though in high fat but this is saturated fat which does not pose any risk. It helps to increase the level of vitamin E in the plasma and red blood cells. The vitamin E and riboflavin are essentially alkalinized. Almonds increases the level of antioxidants in bloodstream, reduces blood pressure and improves blood flow.

Some Other Alkalizing (Or Neutral) Foods and Beverages That Can Be Incorporated

This includes soy, such as miso, soy beans, tofu, and tempeh; unsweetened yogurt and milk; most fresh vegetables; herbs and spices, excluding salt, mustard, and nutmeg; beans and lentils; some whole grains, such as millet, quinoa, and amaranth; herbal teas; and fats like olive oil

Chapter 5

Alkaline Diet

Alkaline diet is a school of thought which postulate the consumption of some specific foods which help the body to be more alkaline in order to protect it against some conditions such as inflammation as well as body weight management.

Foods and drinks that promote alkaline diet are discussed in early chapters of this book. However, alkaline diet practically frowns at taking alcohols and / or caffeine. It also discourages the consumption of dairy foods and processed foods.

As earlier described, a pH level measures how acid or alkaline a substance is where a pH of 0 is totally acidic and a pH of 14 is completely alkaline. A pH of 7 is considered neutral. The body may tend to want to shift here or there which is why the alkaline diet is encouraged. There is the claim, though controversial, that a diet low in acid-producing foods and high in fruits and veggies could help avert kidney stones, keep bones and muscles in good forms, improve the healthy functionalities of heart and brain, ease low back pain and reduce the risk for type 2 diabetes.

When alkaline diet is brought to the fore of one's diet, this goes to say that one has made the choice of fruits and vegetables in the stead of foods and substances higher in calories and fats.

Most or all of our consumptions are either of acidic or alkaline outcome where acidic intakes expose the body to inflammation and disease while alkaline intakes would reduce inflammation and reprove other diseases. Alkaline environment does not give room for diseases.

Inflammation is the way the body responds to injuries and infections. When there is an injury to the body or damage to tissues in the body, via the immune system, the body tries to fight or heal this injury or repair the damaged tissue. This is the description of inflammation and is linked with pains on tissues and joints. When you consume acidic foods then inflammation is aggravated. In similar veins, when alkaline foods are consumed, the body reduces inflammation, for all intents and purposes of eliminating pain and disease.

The process is such that the body works to restore the pH balance in reaction to consuming acidic foods which requires releasing alkaline-rich minerals into the bloodstream.

As it has been submitted here and by many other authors and researchers, the ideal range of pH operational level is 7.0, it is on this that the body operates on a balance of its acidity and alkaline, the scale of which ranges from -4.5 (i.e hyper acidity) through to -9.5 (highly alkaline). To enjoy good health and vitality, it is essential to balance pH level in the body.

In conclusion, for a balanced pH condition, alkaline intakes should be targeted at 80% while acidic intake should be at the maximum of 20%.

Chapter 6

Acidic Diets

Acidic diets refer to food and drinks i.e substances that have pH level of 4 – 6 or lower.

As discussed earlier, the pH value indicates whether something is acidic, alkaline or neutral. A pH of 0 is totally and highly acidic, a pH of 14 is also completely alkaline, and a pH of 7 is neutral. For further explanation, a cell-battery is an example of something that is extremely acidic at pH of 0, pure refined water at pH of 7 i.e neutral (neither acidic nor alkaline, and liquid drain cleaner is at pH of 14 i.e extremely alkaline.

High – Acid Foods and Drinks

The list of foods and drinks on high-acid always attracts controversies among experts.

Examples of Acidic foods

Animal proteins, some legumes, wheat/gluten, sugar, caffeine, alcohol, some particular dairy products, eggs, grains, fish, processed foods, sodas and other sweetened beverages

Fruits and Their pH

Fruits	pH
Lime	2.00 – 2.80
Blue plums	2.80 – 3.40

Grape	2.90 – 3.82
Pomegranate	2.93 – 3.20
Grapefruit	3.00 – 3.75
Blueberries	3.12 – 3.33
Pineapple	3.20 – 4.00
Apple	3.30 – 4.00
Orange	3.69 – 4.34
Peaches	3.30 – 4.05
Tomatoes	4.30 – 4.90

In general, citrus fruits have a low pH, i.e they are acidic. Notwithstanding their initial acidity, most fruits are alkalizing.

Fresh vegetables

In general, vegetables, fresh vegetables especially, are not considered acidic. Below is a list of some vegetables and their pH levels:

Vegetable	pH
Sauerkraut	3.30 – 3.60
Cabbage	5.20 – 6.80
Beets	5.30 – 6.60
Corn	5.90 – 7.50

Mushrooms	6.00 – 6.70
Broccoli	6.30 – 6.85
Collard greens	6.50 – 7.50

Excessive acidity can increase the risk for cancer, problems, and heart disease.

Chapter 7

Making The Body More Alkaline

Going alkaline keeps you healthy, making you feel good and making you look good.

Alkaline diet helps the body not to be acidic thereby preventing lack of energy and feeling bloated. According to science, our health is largely depended on what we eat and how well they are digested. Alkaline diet is a diet that concentrates on handling illnesses that relate to digestive issues. This is due to the fact that digestive system is seen as very important for the maintenance of wellbeing, tissue function, inner health as well as posture. This goes to emphasise the importance of the function of a healthy/alkaline digestive system to the body as it concerns energy level and weight control.

Professionals have postulated that diets that are too acidic can be described as poor eating habits which can lead to bad health.

Making Change

Effecting these changes requires high concentration on consumpt5ion of whole foods such as beans (lentils in particular), fruits, nuts, seeds, spices, vegetables and whole grains. Others are cucumbers, chia seeds, leafy greens, lemons and melons, all of which examples of alkaline producing foods.

Furthermore, instead of caffeine, go for herbal teas like ginger or green tea, take a lot of green juice, and add lemon to alkalized fluid.

It is also advisable to eat smaller quantities of fats, meat, fish, pasta and other types of grains. Always go for high quality oils like olive oil, coconut oil and avocado oil.

Stay away from taking processed foods as well as artificial foods, caffeine, white sugar and white flour.

The reason for the body to be alkaline

Healthy body is influenced by the pH level. Health or body discomfort as mild as fatigue, runny nose, or a skin break could be an indication that the body is too acidic. The way out of this is to concentrate on alkaline foods and supplements in order to bring the body back into shape by increasing the alkaline level in the body. Boosting the alkalinity of the body increases energy level. In order to achieve this, it is advised to focus on consuming foods that are alkaline in nature. In furtherance to the above enumerated foods/drinks, fruits, vegetables, nuts, seeds, legumes, etc are foods that promote alkaline and it is advised for diet to be designed around this.

In similar vein, processed foods and foods like dairy, eggs, and canned foods are acidic and should not be tolerated

About The Author

Lionel Chris is a dedicated and passionate author. Writes on all areas of life – government, health, fitness, economics, business, fiction, poetry and others. Always craving to improve the world through writing and various other natural arts.

Acknowledgement

I have always wanted a platform where I would be able to express some views and share knowledge and experiences. I had imagined different windows to do this without knowing how, where and when to start until I met *Brownie!* Beside putting it down, she is everything about me writing and publishing.

I am eternally grateful to *Kay* for accommodating me to every end that I enjoy.

To everyone at *Apartment I, BA*. All they see in me is a family and relative.

Finally, to TMI, TT, TS and TM. Love you guys.